T0144827

NURSE BARB'S
PERSONAL GUIDE TO
PREGNANCY

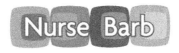

BARBARA DEHN, R.N, M.S.
Women's Health
Nurse Practitioner

Basic Health
PUBLICATIONS, INC.

Basic Health Publications, Inc.
www.basichealthpub.com

Library of Congress Cataloging-in-Publication Data is available through the Library of Congress.

Editor: Carol Rosenberg • www.carolkillmanrosenberg.com
Typesetting: Gary A. Rosenberg • www.thebookcouple.com
Cover design: Jan Davis • www.JanDavisDesign.com
Illustrations by Andrea Kelley

Contents

Introduction

$\mathcal{W}$elcome to the most incredible journey of your life! Pregnancy is a time when your body will change in ways that may be difficult to imagine right now. You may feel overjoyed, worried, elated, and overwhelmed all at the same time. Whether you're newly pregnant or closer to delivery, it's normal and natural to have thousands of questions. As your baby grows, some of what you may be experiencing may be a happy surprise, a little shocking, or a little of both. In any case, this booklet has been designed to help you navigate your way through your amazing journey with the most up-to-date information you need for a healthy and happy pregnancy.

WHAT YOU'LL FIND HERE

This booklet is packed with answers to the most common and pressing questions every pregnant mom has. I've also included information on what to avoid, how to improve your nutrition, advice about sex, tips for every stage of pregnancy, helpful to-do lists, and important warning signs to help you determine when and why to contact your OB provider, doctor, nurse practitioner, or midwife.

In addition, I've added a list of useful websites, a form you can use to track your baby's kick counts, and a list of what to bring to the hospital.

Pregnancy is an adventure that will be filled with joy and surprises. I hope that you and your baby will be healthy and happy. *Enjoy your journey!*

CHAPTER 1

When You First Find Out

*W*hen you first find out that you are pregnant, the question "Is this really happening?" might spring to mind. Many women can't believe that they're really pregnant the first time that a pregnancy test comes back positive, and some will take two, three, or more pregnancy tests before the reality actually sinks in. In case you're wondering, the pregnancy tests that are available over the counter at any pharmacy or drug store are just as accurate as those available from your healthcare provider or clinic.

There's no one "right" way to experience a pregnancy. You may feel elated and delighted by the news, enjoying every aspect as your body changes, your baby grows, and delivery approaches. Or you may feel a little bit unsure and ambivalent. It's normal to have mixed feelings, especially when you first find out. For many women, every moment of their pregnancy is magical; for others, it can be a mixed bag of delightful surprises and difficult challenges.

Your pregnancy and baby will be as unique as you are. What you experience is influenced by numerous factors, including your age, family history, any medical conditions, nutrition, work, exercise, and hormone levels, to name just a few.

IT'S NORMAL TO FEEL OVERWHELMED

Even if they've been trying for months or years to get pregnant, many women feel unsure, scared, and overwhelmed when they see a positive test result. It's normal to have conflicting feelings, especially if you're nauseated or have other challenges in your relationship or with your family. It's also normal to feel guilty if you're not as happy as you thought you would be, or as elated as other people are when you share your news with them.

My Advice

After practicing for over thirty years as a nurse, my advice is to try to let go of any guilt or fear you might be experiencing and give yourself time to get used to the idea of being a new mom and adding to your family. That's why you get many months to prepare for your baby's arrival. If your ambivalence turns into sadness and a feeling of being completely overwhelmed by your situation, do talk to your doctor or midwife.

HOW FAR ALONG AM I?

This is one of the most common questions people have. Most think that pregnancy lasts for 9 months, when actually it's 40 weeks from the first day of the last menstrual period. Though we know that pregnancies don't start on the first day of the last period, it does provide a date to start calculating when ovulation and conception may have occurred, which is usually sometime between 10 and 16 days after the first day of the period.

Pregnancy is 40 menstrual weeks, which means that when a woman is 1 week late for her period, she is 5 weeks pregnant. In reality she's only been pregnant for 3 weeks. Though this can be confusing, everyone around the world calculates pregnancies based on the number of weeks from the last period. If there hasn't been a period, then we use ultrasounds or other ways to determine how many weeks along the pregnancy is.

It's very important to be able to calculate the number of weeks along a mom is in order to determine how the baby is growing throughout the pregnancy, to estimate the due date, and to prepare for the tests that need to be done at certain times. Knowing the number of weeks is also important if a mom goes into labor too early or too late because both situations affect the baby's health.

You'll also want to know your due date and how long you have been pregnant, as that will influence your appetite, how tired you are, when you might expect nausea and queasiness to improve, and many other changes that you will experience. Planning for the future will also be easier when you have a better idea of what your body and your baby will be experiencing week to week and month to month.

CHAPTER 2

Nausea and Morning Sickness

*T*he good news is that not every newly pregnant mom will experience morning sickness, though the nausea in pregnancy can occur any time, day or night, and can last minutes, hours, or all day.

You may be lucky, like one in three pregnant women, and you may not feel queasy, seasick, or unable to eat. However, approximately two out of every three pregnant moms will start to feel nauseated, starting at about 7 to 8 weeks of pregnancy. The nausea and queasy stomach may be mild at first and worsen every few days.

WHY IT HAPPENS

Nausea is caused by the rapid increase in pregnancy hormones and usually improves by the twelfth to fourteenth week. Moms with twins have more pregnancy hormones present in their bodies and may be more likely to experience nausea.

We also know that genetics plays a role. Women with a family history of a mother, sister, or grandmother who suffered from morning sickness are much more likely to also feel queasy in pregnancy. Sorry to say it, but, if you have nausea with one pregnancy, you're likely to have it with all your pregnancies.

Changes in Smell and Taste May Contribute to Morning Sickness

Many women often develop an enhanced sense of smell in early pregnancy. Newly pregnant moms can detect odors that they were never able to before, or find mild odors much stronger and more noxious and disturbing. It's possible for a pregnant mom to smell French fries cooking from half a mile away!

Being able to detect smells more keenly means that a newly pregnant woman can sniff food and tell if it's gone bad, but it also means that any aroma or odor can make her feel more queasy and nauseated, including perfumes, foods that she may have enjoyed in the past, or strong smells from smoking or laundry. This is a surprising result of increasing hormone levels and can lead to avoidance of certain situations or foods.

In addition to changes in the sense of smell, a woman's taste buds may also change in early pregnancy. Now some foods may have a different flavor, or be less appealing, which may lead to food aversions and also to cravings. You may find that you can't even think about certain foods, or that,

NAUSEA AND MORNING SICKNESS

once you prepare something, suddenly you can't eat it. The old clichés about pickles and ice cream really do apply in early pregnancy. Blame it on the hormonal roller coaster and just wait because your food aversions and cravings may change in a few weeks.

HOME REMEDIES FOR MILD NAUSEA

The key is to try to stay hydrated, because once dehydration starts, it can make the nausea even worse and cause food and fluid aversions, where pregnant moms refuse to drink because just the sight and smell of fluids make them gag.

For mild nausea, there are some easy, practical, tried-and-true options to help you feel a little better, or at least well enough to be able to get some fluids and food into your tummy so that you don't become dehydrated. Below are many of the tips I've gathered that have helped thousands of newly pregnant moms feel better. I hope that they'll also work for you.

Try These Proven Strategies for Morning Sickness:

❏ Before getting out of bed in the morning or even raising your head from your pillow, try to eat one or two dry crackers. Once you've been able to swallow them, wait five to ten minutes, then get up slowly.

9

❏ Prevent vomiting by keeping your stomach half-full throughout the day. An empty stomach is not a happy stomach, and you're more likely to vomit if you eat. So help your stomach stay happy by eating small amounts of food throughout the day.

❏ Try a bite or two of something nutritious every half hour. Think of eating small amounts frequently as if feeding your baby every two hours. It doesn't have to be much. A little fruit, a spoonful of yogurt, or a couple of crackers is often enough to keep your tummy happy.

❏ Try eating bland foods, such as breads, rice, potatoes, or tortillas to settle your stomach.

❏ Do not eat large meals on an empty stomach, as these are likely to come right back up.

❏ You don't have to take your prenatal vitamin every day if it makes you queasy. Try taking it at night or a few times a week if you aren't able to eat a balanced diet.

Try These to Settle a Queasy Stomach:

❏ Anything with ginger can help you feel better: ginger cookies, ginger ale, or ginger candy or tablets. If you can't swallow, you can get the same benefit from sucking on them.

❏ Cut up some juicy fruit, such as watermelon or cantaloupe, which will give you both fluids and a little bit of sugar.

❏ Flavored popsicles can help confused taste buds because they're icy and a little sweet.

❏ Try eating small amounts of bland dry foods without butter, spreads, or other toppings, including:

- Melba toast
- Toast or bagel with nothing on it
- Plain tortillas
- Mashed potatoes
- Plain rice
- Crackers

❏ Consider trying acupressure by wearing Sea-Bands. These are small bracelets that apply slight pressure to your wrist and can help ease nausea.

SEVERE MORNING SICKNESS

Some women have such severe nausea and vomiting that they become dehydrated and malnourished and are unable to keep anything down. This is known as hyperemesis gravidarum and needs to be evaluated and treated by an OB doctor or midwife immediately. If you can't keep any food or liquids down, or if you're vomiting for more than six hours, call your OB provider, nurse practitioner, or midwife right away.

To Rehydrate After Vomiting:

❏ The trick to getting in fluids after vomiting is to think like Goldilocks. Don't drink plain water, it's too bland. Don't drink full strength fruit juice, it's too sweet. Instead, try something in between that's just right! Like Goldilocks, not too much, not too little, but just right.

❏ Mix equal parts of water and juice in a small cup.

❏ Try consuming one teaspoon of your water/juice mixture. This will get absorbed well before it ever gets to your stomach and is unlikely to cause vomiting.

❏ Then repeat one teaspoon every five to ten minutes until you've been able to swallow at least six teaspoons, which is one fluid ounce.

❏ Then you can try small sips of the water/juice mixture, making sure to go slowly until you've had at least six ounces.

❏ If you're not able to tolerate the teaspoons of liquid, then it's time to call your OB provider.

Call Your OB Provider:

❏ If you have been unable to eat or drink anything for six hours or longer while you're awake

❏ If you have been experiencing vomiting or diarrhea for six or more hours

CHAPTER 3

Exercise

*I*f you have been exercising regularly prior to becoming pregnant, that's great! Your conditioning, stamina, and strength will help you and your baby in many ways. In addition to being a great way to help your heart, lungs, and muscles get ready for labor, exercise helps keep blood sugar levels lower, helps prevent constipation, improves mood and outlook, and makes it easier to get a good night's rest. Pregnant moms who exercise are also more likely to keep their weight gain in a healthy range and have enough energy for labor.

Exercise in pregnancy is as simple as taking a walk. Don't give up completely if you can't join a gym or don't have the time to do a full hour of exercise. And remember, this is a guilt-free zone, so any exercise is better than none.

I know you're doing the best you can. Try for a ten-minute walk, which is great; anything more you can do is wonderful. Please don't get discouraged if you can't do as much as you'd like to. Every day is a new day, and you might feel better tomorrow.

Just remember that any exercise is good for you and the baby.

GETTING STARTED

If you haven't been exercising it's never too late to start, even when you're pregnant. However, it's best to start off slowly and gradually increase the time and intensity of your exercise.

You don't have to run a marathon to increase your endurance. Walking is just as beneficial and may be safer than running or jogging. To help you get back into an exercise routine, try walking for fifteen minutes at least five times per week. Gradually increase the time you spend walking by five minutes, until you can comfortably walk for forty-five to sixty minutes every day. This will help you feel better in so many ways.

WHY EXERCISE IS IMPORTANT

Walking helps prevent constipation, improves mood, helps you sleep, and helps keep your blood sugar in a healthy range. In addition, walking every day will help you build up the stamina you need to go through labor and delivery, recover faster, and have more energy to care for your new baby.

Most pregnant moms can and should exercise throughout their pregnancy. However, there are physical changes that may affect how you feel with certain exercises. The following are some things to keep in mind as you exercise.

- **Larger tummy.** This changes your center of gravity and can make roller blading, skating, skiing, and other activities more risky, as you're more prone to falling.

- **Loosening in the joints.** Starting at about 28 weeks of pregnancy, a woman's ankle, hip, and knee joints become slightly more relaxed under the influence of the hormone relaxin. This not only helps the hips widen in preparation for the birth, it also causes the knee and ankle joints to be slightly looser, more wobbly, and more prone to injury with hiking, running, or walking. With added weight to carry, the ankles, knees, and hips can start to ache more, especially at night. If you're experiencing some aching, rest is the best way to remedy the situation; however, if the pain is more severe, be sure to discuss it at your next prenatal checkup.

- **Stretched ligaments.** Your growing uterus is attached to the pelvic structure and held up in place by five sets of strong and sturdy ligaments. Without these workhorse ligaments, everything would be drooping and falling. However, as your tummy expands and your baby grows, the ligaments stretch, which may cause lower abdominal pain, soreness, and cramping, especially if you exercise. This is particularly common with exercises where there's a lot of up and down movement in the hips, such as that which occurs with cycling, hiking, jogging, or using an elliptical or stair machine.

You may find that using a supportive pregnancy belt or bellyband will help take some of the pressure off the ligaments.

If you have any sharp pain in your lower abdomen, it's important to talk to your OB provider right away, so that they can evaluate exactly what it is.

- **Your heart works harder.** As pregnancy progresses, your heart and blood vessels will adapt and grow to keep up with the increasing needs of your baby and your body. Not only does the amount of blood increase, your heart muscles also expand to keep pumping plenty of oxygen-rich blood to the baby and throughout your tissues and organs. That means that your heart is already working slightly harder than it did before your pregnancy.

  Something as simple as climbing a set of stairs or traveling to a place at a higher elevation can cause you to feel slightly out of breath. It's normal and natural during pregnancy to modify your exercise to a lower intensity. It's better to work out a bit longer and at a slower pace than to push yourself to work out at a high intensity. Make sure you listen to your body and slow down if you need to.

- **You may sweat more.** In pregnancy, because you're carrying more weight and your heart is working harder, you may find that you sweat more with exercise.

It's important to stay hydrated and get plenty of fluids all the time in pregnancy and especially when you're exercising. Carry extra water and take more breaks.

Remember, it's better to walk for an hour at a moderate pace than to push yourself to run a mile in under seven minutes. Just as you're nurturing your baby, take care of yourself; stay hydrated with lots of fluids, decrease the intensity of your workout, and remember that any exercise is beneficial for you and your baby.

Depending upon the type of exercising you've been doing, it's likely your OB provider will recommend that you continue. It's also likely that they may ask you to make some modifications if you're into kickboxing, martial arts, rock climbing, or other forms of exercise.

Exercise Guidelines:

❏ Exercise is important, unless your OB provider has advised against it.

❏ Don't exercise if you're bleeding, have premature contractions, or have been advised not to by your OB provider.

❏ If you find yourself out of breath, then decrease the intensity of your exercise.

❏ You sweat more during pregnancy, so be sure to drink plenty of fluids.

❏ If you're exercising outside when it's sunny, be sure to use sunscreen as pregnancy hormones can cause the skin to develop dark spots and more pigmentation on the upper lip and cheeks. These darker areas are known as the "mask of pregnancy."

❏ Work out longer, not harder. Forty minutes of walking at a moderate pace is better than ten minutes of fast walking or jogging, especially if you're out of breath.

❏ After your fifth month, avoid exercising on your back, as the weight of your tummy presses on the big blood vessels that provide oxygen-rich blood to your baby and your body. This position can also lead to decreased blood flow to mom and baby and may cause you to feel lightheaded. If that occurs, simply roll to your side until you feel better, then avoid lying on your back.

❏ Avoid any exercise that could cause you to fall. As your baby grows and your tummy is pushed up and out, your center of gravity changes, and you're more prone to being a little unsteady, tripping, walking into things, or falling.

Recommended	Not Recommended
Walking	Horseback riding
Hiking	Downhill skiing
Swimming	Rock climbing
Cycling	Scuba diving
Yoga	
Low-impact aerobics	

CHAPTER 4

Travel

*S*ome pregnant women travel one, two, or more hours each day commuting to their jobs. Others travel for work or for vacations. Whatever the case, traveling by car, bus, or airplane is generally considered safe for healthy pregnant women. Always consult your OB provider before any extended travel or as your pregnancy progresses into the third trimester.

If you're going to be sitting for an extended period of time, it's best to take breaks every one to two hours by getting up and walking around. Even a quick visit to the bathroom will prevent your bladder from becoming too full and also help with your circulation.

Guidelines for Travel in Pregnancy:

❏ Always wear your seat belt.

❏ It's helpful to place a small pillow at the level of your lower back to provide added lumbar support.

❑ If you're going on a long journey, do bring a pillow for napping.

❑ Drink lots of fluids to stay hydrated, and avoid caffeine.

❑ Pack nutritious snacks and extra water.

❑ Plan for lots of bathroom breaks because most pregnant moms need to use the bathroom much more frequently.

FOR AIRPLANE TRAVEL

It's generally considered safe for healthy pregnant women to fly on commercial airlines. However, if you plan to fly late in your pregnancy close to your due date, or on a flight lasting more than six hours, or in a private plane that is not pressurized, then do check with your OB provider for guidelines. Here are some tips to keep you and your baby comfortable and healthy as you travel by plane:

• Request an aisle seat for those frequent trips to the bathroom.

• Bring an extra pair of loose-fitting shoes in case your feet swell.

• Plan to get up, use the bathroom, and walk around every two hours.

• Drink lots of fluids to stay hydrated, and avoid caffeine.

• Pack nutritious snacks and extra water.

- Make sure you have everything you need in your carry-on bag, in case your luggage gets lost or is delayed.

- Each airline has different rules about how late in pregnancy a woman may fly. You may need a note from your OB provider in your third trimester.

CHAPTER 5

Sex

*M*ost women and their partners have questions about whether they can continue to have sex during the pregnancy. It's normal and natural for both partners to have concerns and questions. It's also normal to be too embarrassed to bring this up with your OB provider, which is why I've included lots of helpful information here. You and your partner may have conflicting feelings about sex. In general, for healthy pregnant women, sex is safe and does not harm the baby.

WHAT'S NORMAL

It's normal for your interest in sex to change as your body changes. Many women have less interest in the first trimester, especially if they feel nauseated and exhausted. Some have more interest as their breast size increases or during the second trimester when their hormone levels change.

It's also normal to wonder if it's safe to masturbate, use a vibrator, or be self-sexual in pregnancy. The same guidelines apply to women who are with a partner as to those who are self-sexual.

RELATIONSHIPS

Partners may feel unsure about whether sex harms the baby, or if their partner is hesitant about sexual intimacy as more of her focus turns away from their relationship and turns inward. Partners often say they feel guilty for wanting to have sex.

Many times in a relationship, one person is more interested and comfortable having sex during pregnancy than the other person is. Couples may experience lots of tension as one person tries to persuade or convince the other that sex is okay and "we can just go ahead," while the other is less interested and may be avoiding sex. It's not always the non-pregnant partner who is more interested. Sometimes a woman's pregnancy hormones increase her sex drive, which can be a happy surprise or add more pressure in the relationship.

One thing is for certain: everything changes in a relationship when a woman becomes pregnant. The most important way to keep the relationship healthy and happy is to find ways to communicate about everything, including sex, with support and love.

It's a lot easier to have sex than it is to talk about it, and yet it's essential for both partners to feel that they are being heard, respected, loved, and supported. That's not always easy to do and can be especially challenging when the woman is pregnant. With hormone levels that are changing, a body that is growing, and a new baby to prepare for, everyone's sexual relationship changes.

No matter if you're more interested in having sex or less interested, you're perfectly normal and natural. The key is to talk to your partner about what will work in your relationship.

It's Normal to Have:

- **More interest in sex:** More blood flow to the pelvic area and larger, firmer breasts may enhance your interest and enjoyment. You may experience more powerful orgasms in the first and second trimesters.

- **Less interest in sex:** Tender breasts, nausea, fear, and fatigue may make sex out of the question for a while.

- **Less fun with sex:** In the last few weeks of pregnancy, as the baby moves down the birth canal, the entire genital area can become much more swollen and uncomfortable. Sex may not be enjoyable and may increase discomfort.

- **Difficulty relaxing:** Most women and men will worry about harming the baby or that the pregnant mom is uncomfortable, which can make it impossible to relax and have fun. If that's the case, find ways to be intimate and close that feel comfortable for both partners.

- **Mixed feelings and thoughts about sex:** It's normal to think and feel differently about sex now that you're pregnant. Open communication is important for your relationship. If you're not able to talk to your partner in a way that feels comfortable, then do talk to your OB provider for some resources and guidance.

- **An interest in new creative positions:** As your body changes, positions that you were comfortable with in the past are no longer possible. Side-lying, having the woman seated on top, or other positions might be more comfortable.

- **A worry about oral sex:** For many couples, intercourse may be too uncomfortable or not part of their intimacy, and oral sex may be more comfortable. For pregnant moms who are receiving oral sex, it's a nice way to be intimate and have fun. Just one important note: partners should *NOT* blow air into the vagina. This can cause a very rare but still serious air embolism, which could affect mom or baby, or both.

You May Feel:

❏ Very sexy and attractive

❏ Guilty

❏ Unsure because the baby is "watching"

❏ Awkward and uncomfortable

❏ Less attractive as your body changes

❏ Hesitant and unable to relax and have fun.

As pregnancy progresses, be creative with position changes and other ways to be intimate together. Gentle hugs or caresses can be a sweet substitute for intercourse. Just as you're nurturing your baby in pregnancy, it's important to feel nurtured and loved by your partner.

Do Not Have Sex if You Have:

❏ Vaginal or abdominal pain

❏ Premature labor

❏ A vaginal or urinary tract infection

❏ Blood or fluid leaking from your vagina

❏ Been advised that you have a placenta previa, where the placenta is over the birth canal

❏ Been advised against it by your OB provider

CHAPTER 6

What to Avoid

*W*hen a woman finds out that she's pregnant, one of the first concerns that comes up is what she should do, and what she should avoid doing, to have the best chance of having a healthy baby. Rest assured that the vast majority of moms and most babies will be healthy, and yet there are some guidelines for what to avoid when pregnant.

WHAT TO STOP

Smoking, alcohol, and recreational drugs— All of these increase the risk of miscarriage, bleeding, smaller babies, premature babies, developmental delays, and other serious complications. Once you know that you're pregnant, it is best to stop them completely.

With alcohol, the concern is having three or more drinks even a few times during the pregnancy, or having a little alcohol every day; these behaviors are considered the most risky. However, the truth is we just don't know how much alcohol is too much for each unique mom and her baby. That's why it's recommended that, in pregnancy, a woman not have any alcohol at all to minimize any possible risk to her baby.

It's very difficult to talk about the challenge of giving up alcohol, smoking, or recreational drugs. There's a lot of shame involved when we think that others may be judging our behavior. If this is your challenge, I encourage you to talk to an OB provider you can trust. They've encountered these situations before, and they will guide you to being as healthy as possible and help you find more resources to decrease or stop the use of these substances.

As hard as these issues are to talk about, it's much better for the baby's health if the people involved in your prenatal and delivery care have a better idea of some of the exposures the baby may have encountered, so that they can better prepare for a baby that may have his or her own health challenges after delivery.

BE AWARE OF DANGEROUS FOODS

Though pregnancy is a time when every mom should try to eat a wide variety of nutritious foods for optimum health, there are some foods that are more risky. During pregnancy, a woman's immune system changes in several ways that enable her to carry the baby and not reject it. That's why her immune system becomes slightly depressed, and she's more susceptible to colds, the flu, and also getting sick from eating certain foods.

In general, pregnant moms tend to have a more severe reaction to exposures to toxins, bacteria, viruses, and other infectious agents than they did before pregnancy. This is because the mom's immune system does not have the same levels of protection it did prior to pregnancy. This makes the mom much more susceptible to becoming very sick from spoiled or contaminated food. In addition, whatever the mom eats may also pass more easily to the baby, who is much smaller and less resistant to toxins or bacteria.

Because a developing baby is so vulnerable to possible harm, it's best to avoid foods that may have high levels of certain chemicals or are more likely to contain bacteria or parasites. The foods on the "avoid" lists in this chapter have all been associated with causing serious harm, including miscarriage. Though you may feel that the risks are slight or have heard conflicting advice, all of these food items have been identified repeatedly as risks for pregnant women.

The confusion can arise because you may hear advice from someone with limited experience and knowledge versus organizations that gather data from thousands of women. My advice when considering the healthiest choices is always use trusted sources of information. When it comes to your health and the health of your baby, there are plenty of other healthy, tasty, and nutritious food options available. Why take the chance of eating something that could be dangerous?

Fish to Avoid:

Avoid these fish that are known to contain high levels of mercury:

❑ Shark   ❑ King mackerel

❑ Swordfish   ❑ Tilefish

Avoid other fish that may contain high levels of PCBs and other industrial pollutants, including:

❑ Striped bass   ❑ Bluefish

❑ Fish from local rivers and lakes that may be contaminated

I recommend SeafoodWatch.org for information about what seafood is safe. You can also check with the Environmental Protection Agency at EPA.org for specific locations and updates on seafood safety.

To be safe, limit all fish, including canned tuna, to less than twelve ounces (3 servings) per week.

Avoid Raw Fish:

If shellfish is cooked properly, it is not considered harmful. However, if fish is raw or undercooked, it could contain bacteria or parasites that are impossible to see and can be harmful to the mom, causing a miscarriage, or causing an infection in the baby.

Do not eat:

- Ceviche
- Sashimi
- Sushi that contains raw fish
- Raw oysters
- Raw clams
- Any other raw shellfish

Other Foods to Avoid:

Because pregnancy goes hand in hand with a slightly depressed immune system and more susceptibility to becoming sick, it's especially important to avoid any risk of acquiring a food-borne illness. The following list of foods may contain bacteria, such as E. coli, listeria, or salmonella, or may contain a parasite, such as toxoplasmosis.

The following foods may cause serious food poisoning or illness in pregnant women and children under five years of age.

Do Not Eat:

- Unpasteurized juice
- Raw meat
- Carpaccio
- Soft cheeses—Even if the label states that it was made from pasteurized milk, these types of cheeses can contain dangerous bacteria.
  - Brie
  - Feta
  - Blue cheese
  - Camembert
  - Goat cheese
  - Gorgonzola
  - Mexican soft cheeses, such as queso fresco

❏ Some deli meats—Salami, liverwurst, and other cured meats may not be made from cooked meats. The slicers at the deli counter may also harbor dangerous bacteria. If you are craving a deli sandwich, ask for it to be heated through or look for something cooked.

❏ Make sure that any hot dogs you eat are also well cooked.

Herbs to Avoid:

Many herbs can be harmful to the baby or can start labor. Please check with your OB provider for more guidance on which herbs should be avoided. This is a partial list of the most common herbs that should be avoided in pregnancy:

❏ Black/blue cohosh or buckthorn

❏ Cascara

❏ Ephedra

❏ Feverfew

❏ Mandrake

❏ Mugwort

❏ Senna

❏ Tansy

❏ Yarrow

Medications to Avoid:

Aspirin and nonaspirin pain medications that contain ibuprofen or naproxen. The latter are also known as NSAIDs (nonsteroidal anti-inflammatory drugs). Aspirin and NSAIDs may cause bleeding or complications for the baby. Tylenol, which is also sold as acetamin-ophen, is generally considered safe. Some-times baby aspirin may be recommended for pregnant women with certain conditions.

Do not take:

❏ Any medication that contains ibuprofen

❏ Motrin

❏ Advil

❏ Nuprin

❏ Any medication that contains naproxen sodium

❏ Aleve

Other Things to Avoid:

❏ **Cats, Cat Litter, and Soil.** I know that you love your cats. However, even if they are indoor cats, their poop may contain toxo-plasmosis, a harmful parasite. Petting and playing with your cat is safe, but changing the cat litter is not. This parasite is airborne, so do not change cat litter while pregnant.

   Toxoplasmosis may also be found in soil or in undercooked beef or pork. When gar-dening, wear rubber or leather gloves and wash fruits and vegetables well. In addi-tion, it's important to cook beef and pork thoroughly.

❏ **Hot Tubs and Saunas.** If your core, internal body temperature gets too high, it can be dangerous for the baby. As moms, we regulate our temperatures by sweating; your baby, however, is surrounded by warm amniotic fluid. It's important to avoid increasing your temperature (and that of the amniotic fluid) by using a hot tub or sauna, which could then increase your baby's temperature.

In addition, avoid soaking in very hot baths where you're completely immersed. If you are sweating, it's likely that your temperature is too high, and it's too hot for the baby. If you want to take a nice warm bath, which can be very soothing for your lower back, be sure that your tummy is out of the water and that you're not sweating.

❏ **High fevers.** If you develop an infection, your core, internal body temperature can get too high, which can be dangerous for the baby. If you have a fever of over 100°F, then call your OB provider for advice.

What to Limit:

❏ **Caffeine:** Caffeine is a stimulant, and some studies have suggested that more than three to five servings a day are associated with an increased risk to the baby. It's probably best to limit your intake to two servings or less each day.

❏ **Artificial sweeteners:** Not enough is known about their effects; however, most experts agree that, because they've been used for years with no known effects, they are probably safe to use.

- **Peanuts:** If you are allergic to peanuts, you shouldn't have them at any time, whether you're pregnant or not. When it comes to preventing a peanut or other nut allergy, we used to think that pregnant women with a family history of nut allergies could prevent their baby from developing an allergy by avoiding peanuts in pregnancy. Recent evidence has shown that this is not the case, and that there isn't a good way to prevent the baby from developing a peanut allergy or other allergy. Unfortunately, peanut and other nut allergies often run in families, regardless of prenatal exposure. The bottom line is, you can eat peanuts as long as you aren't allergic to them.

If you have any other questions about what foods or medications are safe in pregnancy, please consult your OB provider who knows you and your unique situation best.

CHAPTER 7

Lab Tests

*I*n pregnancy, you'll be asked to have many different lab tests. Some are optional and some are standard. These tests will help your OB provider determine how healthy you are and whether there are any concerns for your baby.

STANDARD TESTS IN THE FIRST TRIMESTER

In the first trimester you'll be asked to have several blood tests. These are often ordered after your first visit.

- **Prenatal blood tests:** These test for anemia with a complete blood count (CBC), your blood type, and whether your blood could contain any antibodies that could possibly harm the pregnancy.

- **Blood group and rhesus (Rh) status:** It's important to know what blood group and type you have. This is determined by two factors:

    1. Blood group: People's blood group is categorized as O, A, B, or AB.

2. Rhesus (Rh) status is either positive (+) or negative (–). When a woman is Rh negative and the baby's dad is Rh positive, RhoGAM injections are given to prevent antibodies from forming that could harm this or future babies.

- **Rubella:** Also known as German measles. Most women were vaccinated as children, so they and their babies are not at risk for developing this rare form of measles.

- **Diabetes screening:** You may be tested in the first trimester and/or the second trimester depending upon your risk factors. To screen for diabetes, your OB provider may order a hemoglobin A1c (Hgb A1c) test, a fasting blood sugar, or ask you to drink a glucose solution and then check your blood sugar one hour later.

- **Infections:** There are tests for hepatitis B, syphilis, HIV, and bladder infections. You may also be tested for chicken pox, toxoplasmosis, chlamydia, gonorrhea, and TB.

- **PAP smear:** Tests the cervix for precancerous and cancer cells. This test is often combined with a test for the presence of the high-risk types of human papillomavirus (HPV). If a woman has an abnormal pap smear or high-risk HPV, further testing may be recommended.

- **First trimester ultrasound (U/S):** Your OB provider may perform an ultrasound during your first prenatal visit or order one for you. This first ultrasound looks

NURSE BARB'S PERSONAL GUIDE TO PREGNANCY

for a beating heart and measures the size of the fetus, which is used to determine how far along the pregnancy is and establishes an accurate due date.

In the first 12 weeks, a vaginal probe is often used to provide the best view. It sounds scary, yet it is perfectly safe and painless. In addition to measuring the size of the growing fetus and checking to make sure that the heart is beating, this ultrasound also can be used to measure the baby's neck fold thickness, known as the nuchal translucency (NT), which provides information about the likelihood that Down syndrome could affect the baby.

A first trimester ultrasound is also used to determine if a woman has a tubal or ectopic pregnancy or is having a miscarriage. A woman may or may not have bleeding, cramping, or pain with an ectopic pregnancy or miscarriage.

Miscarriage

Unfortunately, about one in five pregnancies will end in miscarriage. This can be devastating, and it may take a while to recover, both physically and emotionally. Women who miscarry will need to discuss their options for treatment with their OB provider. If you're reading this and have experienced a miscarriage, please do take care of yourself and take the time you need to heal. One miscarriage does not increase the risk of more in the future.

- **Genetic carrier testing:** Based on your ethnic background or family history, you may be offered a test to determine if you are a carrier of common genetic conditions, such as cystic fibrosis, Tay-Sachs, spinal muscular astrophy (SMA), or sickle cell disease. The mother is tested first. If she is positive, then the baby's dad is tested. Carriers of a disease don't show any signs of the disease. Only when both parents are carriers is there a chance of having an affected baby.

STANDARD TESTS IN THE SECOND TRIMESTER

- **AFP/quad screen:** This test is performed between 15 and 20 weeks and is most accurate between 16 and 18 weeks. This screening test analyzes pregnancy proteins and hormones to help find babies who may have a spinal cord or neural tube defect (NTD). About 90 percent of babies with a NTD are found with the AFP/quad screen. This test may also be used, in addition to other blood tests in the first trimester, to screen for serious genetic conditions including Down syndrome (trisomy 21), Edwards syndrome (trisomy 18), and Patau syndrome (trisomy 13). The AFP/quad screen is approximately 90 percent reliable in assessing for these genetic conditions.

As newer, noninvasive prenatal genetic testing (NIPT) becomes more prevalent, the

AFP/quad screen will *not* be used to screen for genetic conditions but will still be used to screen for neural tube defects. If the AFP/quad screen is positive, then further diagnostic testing with ultrasound and amniocentesis is recommended as amniocentesis has a 99 percent reliability rate.

- **Level 2 ultrasound:** This ultrasound is usually performed after 18 weeks of pregnancy. In addition to measuring the baby's growth, the brain, spinal cord, facial structures, limbs, heart, stomach, and kidneys are evaluated. Often the baby's sex can be determined. This ultrasound helps detect the most serious and common conditions that could affect the baby but cannot detect every possible problem.

- **Diabetes screening tests:** These test for gestational diabetes (diabetes that occurs in about 8 percent of pregnancies). A hemoglobin A1c (HgB A1c) test and a fasting glucose test in the first trimester may be followed by a one-, two-, or three-hour glucose tolerance test. If these tests are positive, the mother has gestational diabetes and will need to see a nutritionist and a diabetes educator to help her keep her blood sugar levels in a healthier range. Gestational diabetes is usually controlled by following a specific diet, testing blood sugar several times each day, and by getting regular exercise. Some pregnant women with gestational diabetes will also need to use medications and/or insulin to control their blood sugar levels.

STANDARD TESTS
IN THE THIRD TRIMESTER

- **Anemia screening test:** As your pregnancy progresses and both your baby and your body grows, there's an increased need for more and more blood cells that carry nutrients, calories, and oxygen to the muscles and tissues. Many women can become anemic (a lack of healthy red blood cells) in pregnancy as their body tries to make enough blood cells for the added demands of pregnancy. The body needs iron to make red blood cells, and many moms may need to take more iron to build more red blood cells that can keep up with the increased demands of her growing baby and her growing body. In the third trimester, most moms will have a blood test for anemia.

- **Antibody screening:** Antibodies are our body's natural immune reaction to *any* exposure to something that's different or unknown. Though antibodies develop very rarely in pregnancy, they can occur if there was any bleeding, or if the mom's and baby's blood supply come into contact with each other. Your OB provider will double check for the presence of any antibodies with a blood test.

- **Group B strep culture:** This checks for the presence of the group B streptococcal bacteria, which can be very dangerous to a newborn baby. Because these bacteria (group B strep) can occur in approximately 20 to 35 percent of women without causing any symptoms, this culture is obtained from women close to the time of delivery. For this test, a swab of the vaginal and rectal canals is obtained between 35 and 37 weeks. In a few rare cases, infection with this type of bacteria can cause serious harm to the baby. Less than 1 percent of women who have group B strep will have an affected baby.

OPTIONAL TESTS
FOR GENETIC CONDITIONS

Other tests may be offered or recommended to assess for genetic conditions in the pregnancy. There are differences and trade-offs with the different types of optional tests. Noninvasive tests are screening tests, have no risk of miscarriage, but are not considered diagnostic as they have varying levels of accuracy. Invasive tests, while having low risks of miscarriage, do have higher levels of accuracy and are diagnostic.

Noninvasive Tests

Noninvasive testing means that there's no risk of harming the pregnancy or causing a miscarriage because only the mom's blood is tested.

- **NIPT (noninvasive prenatal testing):** Using a sample of blood from the mother as early as the tenth week of pregnancy, the baby's DNA can be analyzed to detect Down syndrome (trisomy 21) and other serious genetic conditions, including Edwards syndrome (trisomy 18) or Patau syndrome (trisomy 13). There are several good reasons to have NIPT. It has a very high reliability of over 99 percent, no risk of miscarriage, and the rates of false positives are very low at less than 0.1 percent.

NIPT analyzes the cell-free DNA from the baby that's present in the mom's blood supply. This screening test is often recommended instead of using combined and integrated screening, which relies upon several different ultrasounds plus blood tests at different times in the pregnancy and has lower accuracy levels and higher false positive rates.

- **NT (nuchal translucency):** Between the eleventh and fourteenth weeks of pregnancy, an ultrasound is used to measure the baby's neck (nuchal) fold thickness. It's normal for babies to have some fluid in that tiny space; however, too much fluid could be an indicator of Down syndrome. Accuracy is only 60 to 80 percent when using only the NT ultrasound.

- **Combined screening:** This is better than using only the NT ultrasound, as it also adds more information from a blood test that measures pregnancy proteins at 10 to 14 weeks. When both the blood test and the results from a NT (nuchal translucency) ultrasound measurement are combined, the accuracy of the test results is approximately 85 percent to assess the risk of Down syndrome (trisomy 21) and Edwards syndrome (trisomy 18). An accuracy rate of 85 percent means that there is a relatively high false positive rate of 15 percent.

- **Combined integrated screening or sequential screening:** In order to improve accuracy in screening, this test adds an additional test to the combined screening described above. With combined integrated or sequential screening, the results from the combined screening done at 10 to 14 weeks and the NT ultrasound are added to the AFP/quad test done at 15 to 20 weeks.

  By using ultrasound, plus blood tests in both the first and second trimester to screen for genetic conditions, the accuracy rate can be increased to 90 to 95 percent with a 5 percent false positive rate. The downside to these tests is that they take weeks to complete, and a positive test result may lead to the recommendation that an amniocentesis or CVS (see below) be done as a diagnostic test. Both of these additional tests are invasive with a slight risk of miscarriage.

Why We Care about Reducing False Positive Results

When a mom has an optional screening genetic test, it's important to understand that if the test is positive, then she will be asked to have more testing to confirm whether she has an affected baby. Even with a positive screening test, there's still a high likelihood that the baby is healthy and not affected. Unfortunately, having a positive screening test causes a lot of worry and anxiety, and the added testing that's recommended is much more risky for miscarriage. In addition, the mom has to go through all of the emotional trauma of worrying about the baby being healthy, plus she also has to consider having a test that could cause the loss of what could be a healthy pregnancy. That's why it's important to consider noninvasive screening tests, such as NIPT, with low rates of false positive results.

Invasive Testing

Chorionic villus sampling (CVS) and amniocentesis are the most accurate genetic tests available. They are used to assess the chromosomes present in either the developing placenta, which is known as the chorionic villus, or in the amniotic fluid, to diagnose genetic conditions with a better than 99 percent level of accuracy. The trade-off is that, though they are highly accurate, they may lead to the loss of a healthy pregnancy in approximately 1 in every 300 to 500 procedures.

- **CVS:** This is a diagnostic and highly accurate test for genetic conditions, and is

NURSE BARB'S PERSONAL GUIDE TO PREGNANCY

performed at 10 to 12 weeks into the pregnancy. This may be offered to a woman simply based upon her age, if she is thirty-five years or older. Or it may be offered if there was a positive result from a nuchal translucency (NT) ultrasound or NIPT.

Guided by an ultrasound, a specially trained physician will insert a small catheter through the abdomen or vagina to obtain a sample of cells from the chorionic villi. These are the cells that will develop into the placenta. The cells are analyzed for genetic conditions and the baby's sex can be determined. A CVS is 98 to 99 percent accurate in diagnosing Down syndrome (trisomy 21) and other common genetic conditions including Edwards syndrome (trisomy 18) and Patau syndrome (trisomy 13).

With CVS, very rarely, the cells cannot be analyzed with the highest level of certainty. In those cases, which occur 1 to 2 percent of the time, the results are reported as being ambiguous, and further testing may be recommended.

A CVS can also determine whether a pregnancy is affected by sickle cell disease, some types of muscular dystrophy, cystic fibrosis, Tay-Sachs disease, and other rare genetic conditions. It cannot detect every possible health condition in a pregnancy. The miscarriage rate for CVS testing is approximately 1 in 200 to 1 in 300.

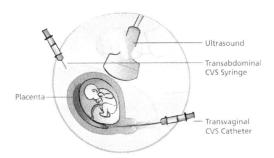

Ultrasound

Transabdominal
CVS Syringe

Placenta

Transvaginal
CVS Catheter

With CVS, either a syringe or catheter
is used to obtain the cells, not both.

- **Amniocentesis:** This highly accurate diagnostic test is best performed between
  16 and 20 weeks. Amniocentesis is often
  offered to women who are thirty-five or
  older for genetic testing, or it may be recommended if there was a positive result
  from one of the noninvasive tests.

  The amniotic fluid is sampled because
  it contains the baby's skin cells, which
  contain the genetic material necessary to
  accurately perform an analysis. Specially
  trained physicians use an ultrasound to
  locate a large pocket of amniotic fluid
  to sample. A needle is inserted into the
  mother's abdomen to withdraw a small
  amount of the fluid.

  Don't worry—the baby and the placenta will make more amniotic fluid, and
  the tiny hole from the needle will heal
  on its own within a few days. The baby's
  sex can also be determined from an
  amniocentesis.

  Amniocentesis is over 99 percent accurate in diagnosing Down syndrome (trisomy 21) and the other most common genetic conditions, including Edwards syndrome (trisomy 18) and Patau syndrome (trisomy 13).

Though amniocentesis can also determine whether a pregnancy is affected by sickle cell disease, some types of muscular dystrophy, cystic fibrosis, Tay-Sachs disease, and other rare genetic conditions, it cannot detect every possible health condition in a pregnancy.

The amniotic fluid is also tested for levels of alpha-fetoprotein (AFP), which is an indicator of neural tube defects. There is a greater than 99 percent accuracy rate. The risk of miscarriage is between 1 in 200 and 1 in 500.

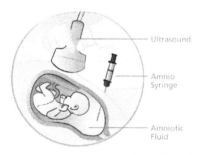

Ultrasound

Amnio Syringe

Amniotic Fluid

Amniocentesis is generally offered between 16 and 20 weeks of pregnancy.

CHAPTER 8

FIRST TRIMESTER
From 1 to 12 Weeks

*F*rom the minute you find out that you're pregnant until the end of the third month, your body will begin to change in countless ways to help nourish your growing baby. You may be surprised by the physical changes that seem to affect every aspect of your life. Emotional changes are also normal and expected. Many women feel as if they're on a hormonal roller coaster.

YOUR BODY

- **Fatigue:** You may be sleeping and waking at odd hours. You may feel exhausted after a normal day at work or find that you're sleeping all weekend. This usually will improve by the twelfth week; in the meantime try to rest whenever you can.

- **Bloated:** Your tummy pops out; your clothes are tight. This is due to water weight gain and the pregnancy hormones, not the baby's growth just yet.

49

- **Constipation and indigestion:** Your intestines slow down to absorb more nutrients and water to help you provide healthy nutrition for your body's and your baby's added needs. Try increasing your fluids, fresh fruits, and veggies. For indigestion or gas, try three chewable papaya tablets after meals. If you're constipated, do talk to your OB provider for advice, as this condition tends to get worse throughout the pregnancy.

- **Cramping and pelvic pressure:** It's a scary feeling. Your uterus is expanding slowly and may cause cramps similar to those experienced during menstruation. Feeling light amounts of pressure in and around the pelvis is also very common. However, if you are doubled over in pain, call your OB provider.

- **Tender and swollen breasts:** You may wonder where you got these new breasts, seemingly overnight. Your pregnancy hormones are helping your breasts get prepared for breastfeeding. The breasts grow and stretch in size. They can feel heavier and more firm, and the nipples can be very tender.

  A good support bra helps support the added weight and may help reduce shoulder and back strain. Look for one that has a wide back strap that's at least 2 to $2^1/_2$ inches wide, and one that has good shoulder support. If you are exercising, be sure to wear a sports bra with enough support so you're not in pain after a workout.

- **No appetite, food aversions, enhanced sense of smell:** Some foods are appealing, while others may make you feel sick. Blame the pregnancy hormones! It's normal to have cravings for certain foods and to be turned off by others. Listen to your body and try your best to eat a well-balanced diet if you can each day. If you're struggling with nausea and vomiting, see my tips and advice in Chapter 2.

- **Frequent urination:** This is normal; it's caused by your growing uterus pressing on the bladder. You may feel as if you have to visit the bathroom every hour. This sensation usually improves after 12 weeks, when the uterus grows out of the pelvis and doesn't press on the bladder as much. If you have any burning or pain when you urinate, do call your OB provider as this could be a sign of a bladder infection.

YOUR EMOTIONS

- **Energized, elated:** Perhaps you're overjoyed with the news and it's all you can think about. You may have dreamed about this and now that it's real, you can't help smiling to yourself. You may be making lists of all the things you can't wait to do with the new baby you'll be welcoming into your life in a few months.

- **Ambivalent:** "How did this happen?" "I'm not ready." It is normal to have mixed feelings and to not be 100 percent sure that this is exactly what you want right now. You're not alone in how you feel; many have felt the same way. It's normal to feel guilty if you're not happy and then to feel many conflicting emotions. Becoming a mom is a huge transition in anyone's life; that's why you get nine months to prepare. So just take it day by day and understand that you'll get more used to the idea over time. If you're really struggling with your feelings, do talk to your OB provider because they can help you.

- **Fear:** It's normal to have concerns about all of the upcoming changes in your body, your relationships, the future, and the health of your baby. Many moms have lots of fears about everything and some don't. Both experiences are normal; different people adjust and cope with the transition to becoming parents in different ways. Do write down your fears and talk about them with your OB provider so that they can help reassure you.

- **Distracted:** With the rush of new hormones, fatigue, and concerns about the pregnancy, many women suddenly feel that it's difficult to concentrate and focus. This is perfectly normal and natural and typically gets better in the second trimester.

- **Overwhelmed:** The amount of information, the advice, and the number of decisions you're confronted with during pregnancy can be overwhelming, especially if you're tired and feeling nauseated.

My Advice

Managing pregnancy is one of the most vulnerable times in a woman's life. Finding an OB provider you can trust and getting prenatal care will help you feel more empowered and in control.

Just remember that you have about nine months to get used to the idea of becoming a mom. There's no one right way to become a mother and care for your child. This is your own personal journey and you are the expert for you. You'll learn a lot about yourself as your pregnancy progresses and as you transition to your new role as a mom and as your family expands to welcome your child. You'll find out what's important to you and what you can let go of. You'll also learn that what works for your friends may or may not work for you. Take the time you need to get the information that will help you make the best decisions for you and your baby.

If You're Overwhelmed

If you're feeling sick, tired, and overwhelmed, remember that you're in *survival mode* right now. Just do the best you can and don't feel guilty.

YOUR BABY

In the first 12 weeks, there is incredible growth and development as a single microscopic cell develops into a growing baby. Your baby's development follows this pattern:

- **6 weeks:** The heart has developed and is now beating. The eyes are developing, are very large compared to the rest of the face, and are closed. The tiny limb buds, which will grow to be arms, legs, feet, and hands, are forming. The developing baby is only $1/4$ inch long—about the size of a peanut.

- **8 weeks:** At this stage, the hands and feet are webbed while the fingers and toes grow longer. All of the major organ systems including the stomach, nervous system, and brain are developing. The baby is about $1/2$ inch long—about the size of a kidney bean.

- **12 weeks:** Now the hands and feet have lost the webbing that connected them and we can count the individual fingers and toes. The baby's sex was determined at conception when the egg and sperm each provided chromosomes; however, now the genitals have grown and developed enough to be visible. The baby is $2^1/2$ inches long now—about the size of a small lime.

NUTRITION ADVICE FOR THE FIRST TRIMESTER

Your baby is teeny tiny and will take from your body what it needs to grow and develop. Make sure that you're supplying your body—and your baby—with all the best and healthiest nutrition you can so that you and your baby will thrive during pregnancy.

- **Prenatal vitamins:** If possible, try to take your prenatal vitamin every day. Many women find that taking it before bed decreases their nausea and upset stomach. Do the best you can, which may mean only taking it every other day. If you're not able to take your prenatal vitamin at all, then do talk to your OB provider for specific advice.

- **Eat every two to three hours:** Eat small, healthy snacks or half-sized meals more frequently to keep your blood sugar levels stable, prevent headaches, and decrease nausea. Your baby is tiny and needs very little now. If possible, try to eat a balanced diet with three to five servings of fruits and vegetables each day.

- **Graze:** Many newly pregnant moms can't even think about eating an entire meal. Instead, graze and have little bites or sips of food throughout the day. Fruit, nutritional bars, crackers, small pieces of cheese, sips of milk, bites of sandwich, teaspoons of rice, or small sips of drinkable yogurt are worth trying.

- **Even when you're not hungry:** Try to feed the baby every few hours. This will help you feel better and keep up your energy level. It's also a good reminder to stop whatever you're doing and take care of yourself right now.

- **Increase your fluid intake:** Drink at least six glasses of water per day. Avoid soda and fruit juice, as these add empty calories and will fill you up.

First Trimester To-Do List:

❏ Have your prenatal lab tests.

❏ Arrange genetic counseling. This provides an assessment of the likelihood of your having a child with a genetic condition and is an opportunity to discuss the risks, benefits, and limitations of all your prenatal testing options, including NIPT, combined screening, CVS, and amniocentesis.

❏ Ask your provider about NIPT. This is a noninvasive blood test that helps determine the risk of common genetic conditions such as Down syndrome.

❏ Look into cord blood banking with Cord Blood Registry (CBR).

❏ If you decide to have CVS. Schedule the test between 10 and 12 weeks and arrange to have your blood work first.

❏ Keep a journal. Writing down how you feel and the changes you're experiencing is fun to re-read after your baby arrives. You can also write letters to your baby with your hopes and dreams for your future family.

❑ **Call your insurance company.** See what's covered, what's not, where you can have lab work performed, and where you can deliver your baby. Finding out whether you have a copay and what it will be will help you budget accordingly. Now is not the time for financial surprises.

❑ **Try to rest as much as possible.** Your body is creating a baby. That requires a lot of energy! Don't be surprised if you are tired when you wake up and that you crave a nap by 3:00 PM. It's normal to feel fatigued, so listen to your body and nap when you can.

❑ **Discuss your risk of preterm birth with your OB provider.** About one in ten babies is born early; it's best to know your risks and the signs of preterm labor, as well as testing and treatments that are available to reduce your risk.

❑ **Try to exercise.** If you have the energy, try walking at a relaxed pace for twenty to forty minutes each day, or see the guidelines on exercise in Chapter 3. Exercise helps combat fatigue, improves mood and your overall sense of well-being, and helps with constipation.

❑ **Have a good sense of humor.** This helps with all the body changes that are completely out of your control.

❏ **Sign up for a prepared childbirth class.** These and other parenting classes can fill up early, so sign up as soon as possible.

Call Your OB Provider

❏ If you are bleeding.

❏ If you have a severe headache.

❏ If you have severe abdominal or pelvic pain.

❏ If you have had vomiting or diarrhea lasting more than twelve hours.

❏ If you have a fever of over 100°F.

❏ If you have any concerns.

CHAPTER 9

SECOND TRIMESTER
From 12 to 28 Weeks

*T*his is the fun part of the journey. By now, you're probably getting a little more used to the amazing and surprising changes in your body. You're feeling better, and there's less nausea and fatigue. Now you've got more energy, have a healthy radiance, and look great! Is it the glow of pregnancy? You bet it is!

YOUR BODY

In the second trimester, most moms are sleeping better, have an increased appetite, and have lots more energy. At 12 weeks, you'll notice that you have a little tummy showing and that it's time to buy some new clothes, and by 28 weeks there's little doubt that you're expecting, as you have a very obvious pregnant tummy.

As the baby grows inside your uterus, it will take up more and more space inside your abdomen, causing pressure on the bladder and other organs. This comes hand in hand with external signs of your baby's development, such as:

- **Stretch marks:** Your skin will stretch as your tummy enlarges. This may cause some itching or reddish marks. Try to keep the skin moisturized as much as possible with any lotion, cream, coconut, or other body butters; they all work about the same and so you don't need to spend extra money to get the same results. You can also try wearing supportive underwear or bike shorts to help support the weight of your growing tummy.

- **Baby's movement:** You may feel the baby move as early as 18 weeks; however, most moms will feel movement regularly by about 23 weeks.

- **Some difficulty with breathing is expected now:** As your body changes and your baby grows and develops, your body will adapt by making more blood. In addition, your heart will enlarge slightly to pump the extra blood. Now that you're carrying a little extra weight, it's normal to feel a bit tired or winded from something as simple as walking, exercising, or climbing stairs. Take your time, which allows your body to adjust slowly. If you live at high elevations, you may also notice that you're becoming winded with very little exertion. Listen to your body, don't push yourself, and allow for extra time if it's needed.

- **Bleeding gums may occur:** It's normal for your gums to swell and bleed from the increased hormones your body is producing. This is known as pregnancy gingivitis and means that the gums may also feel a little bit sore or tender. Be sure to brush and floss regularly, try a soft toothbrush, and continue to see your dentist. If there's heavy bleeding, check with your OB provider or dentist.

- **Varicose veins:** The added pressure from your growing baby can make it more difficult for the blood in your legs and feet to return to your heart. The blood vessels that carry the blood may stretch and expand causing varicose and spider veins. To prevent this from becoming worse, avoid crossing your legs, try wearing support stockings, and put your feet up whenever you can.

- **Skin changes:** You may be surprised to see a return of teenage acne on your face, back, or chest from hormonal changes. This is one of the changes in pregnancy that no one ever reveals. You may also notice darker pigmentation on your face, especially around the upper lip and cheeks. This is known as the mask of pregnancy, or melasma, and can get quite dark. It's a normal process, but can change your appearance. It's recommended that you continue to use sunscreen during pregnancy, which may help prevent more noticeable darkening.

- **Ligament pain:** These are small twinges or side aches that you may feel when walking up a flight of stairs, exercising, or getting out of bed. These are normal and occur because the baby is growing so much inside your uterus, which in turn stretches the supporting ligaments that hold the uterus in place. Slight twinges are normal and expected. However, if you're doubled over in pain or your pain seems more severe, do call your OB provider.

- **Contractions:** It's normal to feel two to four mild contractions each day now. These are often called Braxton Hicks contractions and seem to be your body's way of practicing for labor. A few contractions each day is not dangerous or a sign of labor. However, if you have three, four, or more contractions in an hour, call your OB provider right away as you will need to be evaluated for premature labor.

- **Anemia:** It's very common to develop anemia in pregnancy from the added needs of both your body and your baby. If anemia is diagnosed, you will need to take extra iron. Try eating more red meat, green leafy vegetables, eggs, and beans, which are all high in iron. If you need to take an iron supplement, they are best absorbed with fruit juice, not with milk. Taking iron can cause constipation, so increase your fluids, fiber, fruit, and vegetable intake.

YOUR BABY

- **12 weeks:** Though she's still only as big as a small lime at 2 inches long and weighs approximately $1/_2$ ounce, all of her organ systems, including the brain, heart, lungs, stomach, and kidneys are rapidly maturing and growing. Her muscles and bones will now grow much more rapidly.

- **16 weeks:** In just one month, he has doubled in length to be over $4^1/_2$ inches long. Now he weights $3^1/_2$ ounces and is the size of an orange. His ears are developing enough to be able to hear you and now he has eyelashes and fingernails. His arms and legs are getting longer and his fingers can open and close. He may even start sucking his thumb.

- **20 weeks:** She is covered with fine hair, called lanugo, and spends a lot of time sucking and swallowing the amniotic fluid that surrounds her. Now you'll probably be able to feel her movements because she weighs almost 1 pound and is 7 inches long, about the size of a banana.

- **24 weeks:** Your baby is about the size of a small melon now, and he has started to follow his own growth curve. He may be 10 to 12 inches long. At this point a baby's weight can be 12 to 20 ounces. His eyes start to move, though they are still closed. As his body prepares for delivery, his lungs continue to develop and produce surfactant, which is essential for breathing air. His skin is thin and see-through. If he is born now, he will need to spend time in a neonatal intensive care unit (NICU) to continue his growth and development.

- **28 weeks:** By the end of the second trimester, she may be 13 to 15 inches long and weigh 1 to 2 pounds. Her skin becomes less see-through and even a little wrinkled. As she prepares for birth, she will practice breathing movements. Now her eyes open and close. A healthy infant who is born now has a good chance of survival and will need to stay in a NICU to continue growing and developing.

NUTRITION ADVICE FOR THE SECOND TRIMESTER

In the early part of the second trimester, if your nausea is gone, it's a good time to try to eat a balanced diet. Your baby needs a variety of healthy nutrients to grow and develop, which is why most women have an increased appetite and cravings for certain foods now. You really are eating for two! Most women need to gain 20 to 35 pounds during their pregnancy.

Cravings

In general, it's okay to give in to food cravings, and cravings may be your body's way of telling you that you need certain nutrients. Eating more fruits and vegetables is always a good idea. If you're craving spicy and salty food, or maybe have a more developed sweet tooth, it's okay to give in and enjoy those foods. You're nurturing a new life, so go ahead and nurture yourself. However, if you're gaining too much weight, you may have to limit some of your indulgences and be more moderate.

If you're having cravings to eat nonfood items such as soil, clay, laundry starch, paint chips, or ashes, or to crunch on ice all day, you may have a condition known as pica. Do talk to your OB provider if you're craving or eating these nonfood items because they can be harmful to you and the baby.

Every Day, Aim to Eat:

❏ A prenatal vitamin.

❏ Protein. Three servings per day. Each serving is about the size of your fist.

- Chicken
- Meat
- Fish
- Eggs
- Nuts
- Soybeans
- Beans

❏ Calcium-rich foods. Three servings per day. Each serving of dairy is one cup.

- Milk
- Yogurt
- Cheese
- Cottage Cheese

If you don't tolerate dairy, then try calcium-fortified juice or a supplement. You'll need 1,200 mg per day. These foods also contain some calcium:

- Green leafy vegetables such as broccoli and spinach
- Almonds
- Sardines

❏ **Vegetables.** Aim for three to five servings each day. Lots of color on your plate means you're getting lots of vitamins, nutrients, and antioxidants. Variety is the key, so try to look for yellow, orange, red, and green vegetables. Salads are a great way to get two to three servings at one meal. Snacking between meals on baby carrots, cherry tomatoes, and celery provides lots of healthy nutrients for you and the baby; plus eating lots of vegetables will help keep you feeling full and prevent constipation.

❏ **Fruit.** Have two to three servings per day. It's better to eat the fruit than to drink the juice, because eating whole fruit provides pectin and fiber and helps you feel fuller. Now's the time to try new fruits and add some variety to your routine, by eating different fruits and berries in season; or try cutting up a melon to snack on. Eating fruit will also provide a range of healthy nutrients and vitamins for you and the baby, and as an added bonus helps prevent constipation.

❏ **Bread, cereal, rice, pasta.** Six to nine servings per day. If you're a vegetarian, you'll need to eat twelve to fifteen or more servings of carbs each day. These are important sources of ready energy. Most people eat double to triple the amount that they need each day, which can contribute to too much weight gain. In general, have two servings at each meal and one serving during snacks.

Avoid the simple carbs, like cookies, white bread, and flour tortillas, and aim to eat more complex carbs from whole wheat bread, beans, corn tortillas, cereal, brown rice, potatoes, and pasta. The trick is to make sure you're not eating too many carbs because, besides contributing to too much weight gain, they may lead to developing gestational diabetes (the diabetes that can occur during pregnancy).

One serving of carbohydrates is small and equals:

- 1 slice of whole wheat bread
- $^1/_2$ slice of white bread
- 1 corn tortilla
- $^1/_2$ flour tortilla
- $^1/_3$ cup cooked white rice
- $^1/_2$ cup cooked brown rice
- $^1/_2$ cup cooked beans
- $^1/_2$ cup cooked corn, peas, or green beans
- 1 small potato or $^1/_2$ large potato
- $^1/_2$ cup cooked pasta

❑ Fats and oils. Fats and oils are essential for the baby's brain development. They are packed with calories and energy, which means a little goes a long way. You only need four servings per day. Because a lot of food already contains some fat, it's best to watch your intake. One serving is just one tablespoon of vegetable oil, mayonnaise, butter, or peanut butter.

❏ **Make every calorie count.** Avoid fast or junk food if possible, and whenever possible have salads or vegetables with meals.

When you indulge in your favorite foods and treats, do savor and enjoy them. Let go of any guilt and remember to nurture yourself while you're carrying your baby.

Second Trimester To-Do List:

❏ **Have the AFP/quad screen.** Performed at 15 to 20 weeks.

❏ **Schedule amniocentesis.** If recommended, this is performed between 16 and 20 weeks. This may be recommended if you're over 35 years of age, or if you've had a screening test that needs further evaluation.

❏ **Have a level 2 ultrasound.** Between 18 and 22 weeks; you'll be able to see the baby's growth and development, see all the major organs, and find out your baby's sex.

❏ **Start sleeping on your side.** At 20 weeks, your right or left side is okay as long as you're off your back, because the added weight of the baby can compress the large blood vessels that carry blood to and from your heart to your body and your baby. Sleeping on your side helps the blood return to your heart more easily and helps ease the feeling of being light-headed. Try using a body pillow to help support your legs and growing tummy.

❏ **Take the one-hour glucose test.** At 24 weeks to 28 weeks. This is one of the tests for diabetes.

❏ **Get the RhoGAM injection.** At 28 weeks, if you are Rh negative.

❏ **Start kick counts.** At 28 weeks, babies should move ten times within one hour. You can find a kick count sheet on page 86.

❏ **Think about who you'd like to have with you during labor.** Your partner and perhaps a friend or family member. Some moms may decide to hire a doula, in addition to having support from the hospital nursing staff and their own OB provider. Doulas have training and experience supporting women in labor.

❏ **Learn about Kegel exercises.** They help prevent leaking urine later in the pregnancy (which unfortunately may occur).

❏ **Sign up for a breastfeeding class.** You can download *Your Personal Guide to Breastfeeding* at NurseBarb.com as an additional resource.

❏ **Read a few books.** Learning about pregnancy, childbirth, baby care, and parenting can ease your mind.

❏ **If you're considering cord blood banking,** the number-one recommended bank by OB/GYNs is Cord Blood Registry (CBR).

Call Your OB Provider:

❏ If you are bleeding

❏ If you have a severe headache

❏ If you have any leaking fluid from your vagina

❏ If you have severe abdominal or pelvic pain

❏ If you have a fever of over 100°F

❏ If you have any feeling of pressure or pain that comes and goes three or more times per hour

❏ If you have any concerns in general

CHAPTER 10

THIRD TRIMESTER
From 28 Weeks until Delivery

*Y*our journey may seem harder now. Your tummy is stretched as far as it can go, and yet every day, it grows bigger and bigger. There are many physical changes that may occur now that are difficult or seem overwhelming. It's normal to feel tired and cranky as you get closer to your due date, while at the same time being excited to meet your baby at last.

YOUR BODY

For some of these symptoms, rest and regular exercise are the best remedies. For others, only delivery itself brings relief. If you don't find the symptoms you're looking for, check back in the second trimester section.

- **More clear vaginal discharge:** This is normal and yet may be hard to distinguish from urine and leaking amniotic fluid. If there's any doubt, call your OB provider.

- **Milk from the breast:** You may notice a little milk leaking from your breast, which may or may not happen. It's best not to squeeze the nipples to see if it's coming out, as this can lead to a contraction. It's also normal if you don't see any milk leaking. Neither situation predicts whether you'll be able to breastfeed.

- **Frequent urination:** You may notice that you have to "go" several times each night and multiple times throughout the day. More frequent urination is normal now, as your growing baby and uterus press on the bladder. It's normal to make two to four trips to the bathroom each night. In fact, this may help you learn to function on interrupted sleep so that you are more prepared when your baby comes. If you have any burning or pain when you urinate, call your OB provider.

- **Leaking urine:** No one tells you about this, but it can happen when you cough, sneeze, or laugh. *Ugh!* A little urine leakage is normal as delivery approaches. Try wearing a pad and practicing 50 to 100 Kegel exercises each day. If you're not sure how to do Kegels, then ask about them at your next prenatal visit. If you're leaking and you're not certain that it's urine, or are wondering if it could be amniotic fluid, then call your OB provider right away.

- **Heartburn:** As your baby and tummy grow, they push the stomach up higher toward the rib cage. After a large meal or even as you breathe normally, you may experience heartburn as the acid from your stomach travels up and down the esophagus. Try antacids and eating smaller meals more frequently. Sit up for a half hour after a meal to allow the stomach to empty. When you lie down, try lying on your right side because your stomach empties toward the right and there should be less acid irritating the esophagus.

- **Constipation:** As pregnancy progresses, our bowels slow down to absorb more nutrients, which can result in more constipation. Taking prenatal vitamins and iron can make this worse. Try increasing your intake of water, fresh fruits, and veggies. Exercise can also help get things moving along. Ask your OB provider about using a stool softener or fiber supplement.

- **Hemorrhoids:** Sadly, I'm not kidding about this either. The pressure from your growing baby, plus any pushing with constipation, can lead to swollen, painful hemorrhoids. Ask your OB provider about over-the-counter remedies. It also helps to work on preventing or relieving constipation by eating lots of fruits, vegetables, drinking water throughout the day, and exercising.

- **Skin changes:** Darker nipples and a line down the center of your tummy are normal. You may also notice increased pigmentation on your face. You can continue to use sunscreen safely in pregnancy. See page 60 for advice on stretch marks.

- **Leg cramps:** Cramps may occur in your calves at night and wake you suddenly when you're trying to sleep. These are very sudden, painful cramps that make it difficult to move your legs. Try to point your toes toward your tummy and then back in the opposite direction a few times to work out the cramp. Also, some moms find that increasing their calcium intake from milk, yogurt, or cheese seems to help prevent cramps in the future.

- **Lower back pain and sciatica:** Your center of gravity is changing, and the added weight you're carrying can put a strain on your lower back. You may feel pain in your buttocks or your back that travels down the back of your legs when getting out of bed, climbing stairs, getting out of your car, or after a long day.

  Try these tips: Don't bend at your waist to pick things up; instead try bending at your knees. Don't twist and bend at the same time. Talk to your OB provider about abdominal strengthening exercises and consider seeing a physical therapist for severe pain. You may find that sleeping with a long body pillow can provide enough added support to improve the pain.

- **Swelling face, hands, feet, and ankles:** As pregnancy progresses, many women notice swelling in their faces, hands, feet, and ankles. This is from your body storing up extra water in preparation for delivery. You may find that your rings and shoes no longer fit. As long as you have normal blood pressure and no other symptoms, try getting off your feet as much as possible, elevating your legs, and increasing your water and protein intake. If the swelling becomes painful or severe, discuss this with your OB provider or midwife.

- **Tingling or numbness in your hands:** As your body prepares for delivery, you may notice that your fingers and hands are more swollen and that, in addition to your rings not fitting, you also have trouble making a fist or gripping things. You may also feel tingling or numbness in your hands or drop things because you can't feel them. These symptoms may be signs of carpal tunnel syndrome, which occurs in about 10 percent of pregnant women. Try buying wrist splints at any pharmacy and use them at night to keep your wrists straight. This helps decrease the swelling in the hands and takes some of the pressure off the nerves in the wrists and hands. In any case, do discuss any swelling or pain with your OB provider or midwife.

- **Aching hips:** As the baby prepares for delivery, he nestles into a head-down position in your pelvis. At the same time, your body produces the hormone relaxin, which helps the pelvic bones relax and move apart slightly and widen. This can lead to a sore or achy feeling in your hips, especially at night when you're trying to sleep on your side. This is perfectly normal. Using a body pillow at night may relieve some of the pressure.

- **Difficulty sleeping:** As you get closer to your due date, you may find it nearly impossible to get a good night's sleep from a combination of aching hips, frequent urination, heartburn, and worries about delivery. Many moms can't get comfortable no matter how many pillows they're using. Others have vivid dreams as delivery approaches, which leave them feeling drained in the mornings. If possible, try to nap during the day if you're feeling exhausted. Even if you can't sleep, it's still good to get some rest whenever possible.

YOUR EMOTIONS

- **Mixed feelings:** When you are near the end of your amazing pregnancy journey, it is normal to have mixed feelings about the birth process, meeting your baby, and how you will recover. You may be feeling excited and hopeful and worried at the same time.

- **Protective:** Your body takes up more room now, and it may seem that everyone wants to pat your tummy or give you advice. It's normal to feel protective toward your tummy and your time. You don't have to let others touch your tummy! Unless, of course, you want them to.

- **Tired and irritable:** This is probably due to interrupted sleep and the pregnancy hormones. You may have less patience for family and friends. It's also normal to feel cranky and to cry more easily.

- **Worried:** Every mom worries about delivery. It's normal to be concerned about pain and whether you can get through it, the baby's health, your recovery, and how your life will change with a new baby. If you're feeling very anxious, are crying often, or if the worry is interfering with your life, then talk to your OB provider. These may be early signs of depression, which can continue after the baby is born and lead to postpartum depression. We know that early recognition of depression leads to more successful treatments. You can get more information at Postpartum Support International through Postpartum.net.

YOUR BABY

In the third trimester, babies gain from $1/4$ to $1/2$ pound every week! Each baby is now following their own growth curve. Their organs are maturing and their brains are

undergoing incredible growth as they prepare for life outside your tummy.

- **28 weeks:** At the start of the third trimester, she may be 13 to 15 inches long
  and weigh 1 to 2 pounds. Her skin becomes less see-through and even a little
  wrinkled. As she prepares for birth, she
  will practice breathing movements. Now
  her eyes are opening and closing. A
  healthy infant who is born now and
  those who weigh less than about $5^1/_2$
  pounds have a good chance of survival
  and will need to stay in a NICU to continue growing and developing.

- **30 weeks:** His lungs continue to mature,
  and he has developed patterns for sleeping and waking. His brain continues to
  grow and develop. Now he's 15 to 17
  inches long and weighs between 2 and
  $3^1/_2$ pounds.

- **32 weeks:** She is losing the soft lanugo
  hair on her body and developing more on
  her head now. As she gains more weight
  her skin looks plumper and less thin,
  which will help her stay healthy after
  birth. She is 16 to $17^1/_2$ inches long and
  weighs $2^1/_2$ to 4 pounds now.

- **34 weeks:** You may be feeling his hiccups
  now as he swallows amniotic fluid, a
  good sign of normal development. His
  bones are getting thicker and stronger,
  and now he's 16 to 18 inches long and
  weighs $3^1/_2$ to 5 pounds.

- **36 weeks:** He has snuggled into a head-down position, which most babies will stay in for birth. His brain continues to develop and all of his organs are functioning. He is 17 to 19 inches long and weighs 4 to 6 pounds.

- **By delivery:** Most babies are 18 to 22 inches long and weigh from 6 to 9 pounds.

NUTRITION IN THE THIRD TRIMESTER

Though you may find that your appetite is decreasing, it's important to eat a balanced diet because this is the time when your baby is growing rapidly. It's an especially critical time for the baby's brain development, which is why eating protein at each meal is recommended. In addition, you also need plenty of nutrients, protein, and iron as your body prepares for delivery. See the Chapter 9 discussion on nutrition in the second trimester for more advice and tips.

- Continue taking your prenatal vitamin daily.

- To avoid heartburn and to accommodate your stomach, which is being squished by your growing baby, eat five to six small meals or snacks each day instead of three large meals.

- Avoid carbonated drinks. They make indigestion worse.

- Be sure to eat three servings of protein and calcium each day:

- o **Good sources of protein:** In addition to chicken, meat, and fish, hard-boiled eggs, beans, peas, sunflower seeds, and cashews, almonds, or other nuts are all packed with protein. Try snacking on these or adding them to salads and snacks.

- o **Good sources of calcium:** yogurt, yogurt drinks, cheese, cottage cheese, calcium-fortified juice, sardines, and green leafy vegetables.

Third Trimester To-Do List:

❏ Finalize names, get a car seat, and pack your bag.

❏ Take a hospital tour and choose a pediatrician.

❏ You will have group B strep screening between 35 and 37 weeks.

❏ Arrange for cord blood banking by visiting Cordblood.com.

❏ Discuss expanded newborn screening. These test your baby for a range of serious conditions.

❏ Continue to do your kick counts every day. See page 86 for a kick count sheet to fill in.

❏ Find ways to nurture yourself, whether it's a quick nap or a special outing. Soon you'll be caring for a newborn, and it's important to learn to also find ways to care for yourself.

❏ Keep important phone numbers handy, near your phone, or programmed into your cell phone.

❏ Be sure to discuss when to go to the hospital with your OB provider. Every provider has their own set of guidelines. It helps to keep their instructions handy and have all the important phone numbers for their office and the hospital posted in your cell phone and in your house.

Call Your OB Provider:

❏ If you have a severe headache.

❏ If you have bleeding from your vagina.

❏ If your water bag has broken.

❏ If you have a fever of over 100°F.

❏ If you have decreased or absent fetal movement.

❏ If you see white spots or have any other unusual visual changes.

❏ If you are less than 36 weeks and have any feeling of pressure or pain three to four times or more in an hour.

❏ If you think you're in labor and are having contractions every five minutes or more often.

❏ If you have any questions or concerns.

Enjoy Your Pregnancy!

I hope this booklet has helped you navigate your way through your pregnancy and that you and your baby have a healthy delivery. This is one of the most magical times in your life, and I'm glad that you brought this booklet along for the journey. Good luck and enjoy your little one.

Useful Websites

Babycenter
www.babycenter.com

CBR (Cord Blood Registry)
www.cordblood.com

Babyzone
www.iparenting.com

Fit Pregnancy
www.fitpregnancy.com

Nurse Barb's Daily Dose
www.nursebarb.com

Parenting Weekly
www.pregnancyweekly.com

Postpartum Support International
www.postpartum.net

The Bump
www.thebump.com

WebMD
www.webMD.com

Nurse Barb's Hospital Packing List

For You:

❏ Comfortable and loose clothes to go home in

❏ Two nursing or regular bras

❏ Two to three pairs of underwear

❏ Socks, slippers

❏ Toiletries

❏ Headband or hair ties

❏ Glasses or contacts

For the Baby:

The hospital will provide T-shirts and onesies for your baby; these are the things you need to take them home. In general, babies need an extra layer to stay warm; if you are comfortable wearing one layer, they will need two.

❏ Pack an extra outfit in case they spit up

❏ Two T-shirts or onesies

❏ One pair of pajamas

❏ One sweater or bunting

❏ One blanket

❏ One hat

❏ Car seat

❏ One burp cloth

For Your Partner:

❏ Camera, video camera, extra batteries, chargers

❏ Cell phone

❏ Clothes to sleep in and go home in

❏ Toiletries

❏ Snacks

Other/Miscellaneous:

❏ _____

❏ _____

❏ _____

❏ _____

❏ _____

❏ _____

❏ _____

Notes:

_____

_____

_____

KICK COUNT RECORD

Wk	Day	Start Time	1	2	3	4	5	6	7	8	9	10	Stop Time	Min
28	M														
	T														
	W														
	Th														
	F														
	S														
	S														

Wk	Day	Start Time	1	2	3	4	5	6	7	8	9	10	Stop Time	Min
29	M														
	T														
	W														
	Th														
	F														
	S														
	S														

Wk	Day	Start Time	1	2	3	4	5	6	7	8	9	10	Stop Time	Min
30	M														
	T														
	W														
	Th														
	F														
	S														
	S														

Wk	Day	Start Time	1	2	3	4	5	6	7	8	9	10	Stop Time	Min
31	M														
	T														
	W														
	Th														
	F														
	S														
	S														

Wk	Day	Start Time	1	2	3	4	5	6	7	8	9	10	Stop Time	Min
32	M														
	T														
	W														
	Th														
	F														
	S														
	S														

Wk	Day	Start Time	1	2	3	4	5	6	7	8	9	10	Stop Time	Min
33	M														
	T														
	W														
	Th														
	F														
	S														
	S														

Wk	Day	Start Time	1	2	3	4	5	6	7	8	9	10	Stop Time	Min
34	M														
	T														
	W														
	Th														
	F														
	S														
	S														

Wk	Day	Start Time	1	2	3	4	5	6	7	8	9	10	Stop Time	Min
35	M													
	T													
	W													
	Th													
	F													
	S													
	S													

Wk	Day	Start Time	1	2	3	4	5	6	7	8	9	10	Stop Time	Min
36	M													
	T													
	W													
	Th													
	F													
	S													
	S													

Wk	Day	Start Time	1	2	3	4	5	6	7	8	9	10	Stop Time	Min
37	M													
	T													
	W													
	Th													
	F													
	S													
	S													

Wk	Day	Start Time	1	2	3	4	5	6	7	8	9	10	Stop Time	Min
38	M													
	T													
	W													
	Th													
	F													
	S													
	S													

Wk	Day	Start Time	1	2	3	4	5	6	7	8	9	10	Stop Time	Min
39	M													
	T													
	W													
	Th													
	F													
	S													
	S													

Wk	Day	Start Time	1	2	3	4	5	6	7	8	9	10	Stop Time	Min
40	M													
	T													
	W													
	Th													
	F													
	S													
	S													

Wk	Day	Start Time	1	2	3	4	5	6	7	8	9	10	Stop Time	Min
41	M													
	T													
	W													
	Th													
	F													
	S													
	S													

INSTRUCTIONS

After about 7 months or 28 weeks, most babies will move 10 times within 2 hours. Many will move 10 times in less than 1 hour.

You can easily count your baby's movements by sitting quietly with your hands on your tummy. It's best to avoid any distractions like work, talking on the phone or watching TV. Any movement that you feel counts as a "kick." If your baby seems quiet and isn't moving, have a glass of juice or milk, or try taking a short walk and try again.

Wk	Day	Start Time	1	2	3	4	5	6	7	8	9	10	Stop Time	Min
	M	7:05	✓	✓	✓	✓	✓	✓	✓	✓	✓	✓	7:20	15
	T	8:20	✓	✓	✓	✓	✓	✓	✓	✓	✓		8:30	10
	W													
	Th													
	F													
	S													
	S													

1. Note the time you start.
2. Place a check in the box after each movement.
3. Note the time you stop.
4. Bring this chart to your office visits.

Most babies will move 10 times in about the same amount of time each day.

When to call your provider

- If your baby hasn't moved 10 times within 2 hours.
- You feel less movement than you usually do.
- You have any feeling of pressure or pain that comes and goes 5 or more times in one hour.

Index

About the Author

Barb Dehn, R.N., M.S., N.P., is a women's health nurse practitioner in private practice and a much sought-after television commentator on health issues. She earned a master's degree from the University of California, San Francisco, and a bachelor of science degree from Boston College. Barb is certified as a menopause practitioner by the North American Menopause Society and is a Fellow in the American Association of Nurse Practitioners.

In addition to national appearances on CNN, NBC, and CBS, Nurse Barb, as she is known, took the extraordinary leap of bringing her blog, Nurse Barb's Daily Dose, to national television via ABC television. She is the award-winning author of a series of guides to women's health that are used by millions of women in the United States.

Barb lives in the San Francisco Bay area with her husband and son.

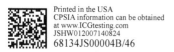
Printed in the USA
CPSIA information can be obtained
at www.ICGtesting.com
JSHW012007140824
68134JS00004B/46